The Widow Coach

Guiding Widows Out of Pain to an Extraordinary Life

By Joann Filomena

Joann The Life Coach
Kingston, New York, USA
Copyright © Joann Filomena, 2017

ISBN: 9781973486749
Imprint: Independently published
Published 2018

DISCLAIMER

Cover Design: Jennifer Stimson
Editing: Maggie McReynolds
Author's photo courtesy of Tamme Stitt Photography

To the beautiful, widowed women who have come through my class for Widow Coaches.
You know that I love you and there's nothing you can do about it!

Table of Contents

Introduction

Dearest Widow,

Since those initial days of shock and the fog encompassing your brain, you've found a way to put one foot in front of the other and get through your day. Maybe you even feel that you are finding some solid footing. It's rocky, no doubt. You have your days when the loss of your spouse is still a raw nerve and everything strikes it. Maybe that's every day for you. Still, you've been moving through your grief and as a matter of fact, friends have sent other widows to you or put you in touch with other widows. You've had coffee with them and were able to make them feel a little better with your shared stories.

That's what a great girlfriend does: She puts her arm around you and commiserates with you. She understands. That empathy can go a long way. It made you feel so great to be doing something to ease the pain for another, even if it was only momentary for her. I hear this from many of you reaching out, even through your own emotional pain, to give solace to another widow. That is how healing begins, for both of you.

But then, it is not enough to be of lasting help to her. You instinctively know it is not, but you don't know how to make a permanent, lasting change in the life of another widow. You want to help more. That feeling of being able to have an impact on someone else's life is so rewarding. But how can you make an even bigger impact, a more lasting impact for her? How can you have a bigger impact in the world?

You get brave. Really brave. You learn the tools that can create lasting change for someone. You learn how to move someone out of the place of emotional pain and teach them to repeat that for themselves, over and over, as needed. This is what life coaching is all about. You hear about it more and more: life coaching. Is it real? What the heck is life coaching? What makes it different than seeing a grief counselor, a therapist, a psychologist?

A therapist, psychologist or psychiatrist works with mental illness. Their client may not even realize they need help. They are able to prescribe medications that can rebalance the chemicals in the brain. They diagnose clients with entrenched problems and treat them long term. They focus on what happened in the past to create the mental issues. They work from the past forward to the present. The therapist will ask the client, "Why and from where did this originate?"

A life coach does not treat, diagnose, or prescribe medication. A life coach works with people who do not have a diagnosis. The life coach's client knows they need help. The life coach focuses on the client's present and helps them improve their future. We are future-focused and solution-focused. Life coaches do not "give advice." As widow coaches, we show the client how to find their own wisdom. We help them reach their full potential in life.

Unless there were pre-existing mental illness issues, a widow is not broken. Grief is not a pathology. Widows are grieving and struggling to re-discover who they are. The widow may be asking what her life is supposed to be now. This is where a life coach can help, and there is no better coach than another widow who has been trained in these tools.

I became a certified, professional life coach after Jim suddenly died. It was the best decision of my life. Through learning to be a life coach, I learned to coach myself. That alone was amazing. But the feeling of being able to focus on work that is making a contribution in the world is my real reward. All my life, I had worked a capital J.O.B. job. It was okay – I did enjoy my work and I didn't need huge rewards from my J.O.B. So much of my life was all about the time spent with Jim and what we explored and learned together. But when Jim passed away, I was left with just a J.O.B. I needed more. I needed growth and the feeling that I could make a difference in the world.

So perhaps that is where you are right now – wanting more from life. With eyes wide open after losing your spouse and suddenly seeing the world for the treasure it really is, you want to make a contribution. You know there is not a second to waste in life. Dear widow, how deeply we truly know this after losing our beloved. This knowledge, this new outlook on the world is what makes us fierce warrior goddesses. We feel like we have just walked through fire.

There are those who devote their lives to actively seeking personal growth, enlightenment, a completely new future for themselves; and they go through the process of trying to shatter their present identity. The seeker who meditates for enlightenment is told to let go of ego completely in order to achieve personal insight and enlightenment. You, dear widow, have gone through involuntary identity shattering. You reached that insight and enlightenment in an instant when your spouse died.

Your ego is a small, quiet voice compared to your previous sense of self. You did not have the luxury of a slow tearing down to slowly rebuild a new sense of identity. You have been thrust right into the fire of rebirth. Now it is up to you how you proceed, if you proceed at all. You can sit in the fire and continue to wonder who you are now. "What do I do now?" we often think. Or you make a choice to begin discovering who you truly are, and even begin to reach for who you can truly become.

I have met many widows – all who, like me, were thrust into the fire of complete destruction of identity. You are no longer a twosome in life, no longer a partner and lover. You had previously built a life and identity together in an equation of two. You became an integral and welcomed part of each other. Suddenly, the earthly bond was broken. The life that was built on an equation of two, stopped. Gone. You are left wondering where to turn. Asking, what's next?

Many of you did the most amazing thing. You eventually looked up from the old easy chair you had been sitting in while mourning, day after day, and envisioned a new life. It was in the power of that new vision or even the singular idea of what could be that drove you to walk forward, reach forward, and start living life again.

So, dear, dear widow, you will continue to carry grief in your heart and you will always remember him and what you had together. But you can also, at the same time, begin to decide who the woman is that you want to become. You can decide that you want to reach out and give a hand up to your widow sisters who are still sitting in the fire.

You've been given the gift of being stripped bare to your soul; now begin creating the amazing, self-aware and fully empowered woman you were always meant to be, and start making a difference in the world. Step forward to become The Widow Coach. Can you really do this? Take my hand. As always, I promise I've got you.

Love, Joann

Chapter 1 – The Widow Journey

It all starts with the journey. I've been in your shoes – just as you stand in mine. It doesn't matter how you came to be widowed. It might have been very sudden, like my own experience. It may have been a lengthy illness. Maybe you had both been told your spouse was terminal. Doesn't matter how – it is always one of the hardest experiences of your life. The post-traumatic stress of losing your spouse to death will mean that in the first six months or so, you are completely removed from reality. Many widows tell me they cannot even remember what happened in those first months. But your brain slowly, slowly begins to ease out of it; leaving you wondering who you are now. What do you do now? You still grieve deeply and feel like this will be forever. Your new normal is this constant series of reminders and exquisite pain. It doesn't have to stay this way. You never give up the love story that was your marriage and your husband. That is yours to keep and treasure forever. But you can begin to see a path before you. It's the path that starts to take you into your next story.

The truth is, that post-traumatic stress and emotional pain is an opportunity for extraordinary post-traumatic *growth*, and there have been studies done and books written to support this. It is the phenomenon that occurs out of the kind of extremely dire circumstances that ignite the human spirit and drive us to not only survive, but to thrive and exceed our wildest dreams in reaching our full potential. Widows often cannot see this. I know. I am the widow coach.

About six months after Jim suddenly died, I was in a new corporate position that had turned ugly. It felt like I was being taken advantage of as a widow. They wanted me to be available and checking in on work seven days a week. Every six weeks, it was required that I cover the "help desk" in the overnight hours (in addition to my regular daytime work with them). It was crazy. I realized I was waking up each morning dreading the work I would be doing that day. This was no way to live my best life. As I sat at my desk, head in hands, I wondered why I was hating the work I had been so happy with for decades. I immediately knew the answer: I used to be able to coach and nurture my team of transcriptionists. I life- coached in the corporate setting for decades. But the ability to track digital data on every employee seemed to have changed corporate America for the worse. Now they just wanted the numbers and demanded I "cut" anyone with low numbers. No checking in to see what was going on with them that might have caused their work to slide. No reaching out to help them refocus and love their work again. All the rewarding, human aspects of my job had gone away.

When Jim was growing up in Queens, NY, he attended parochial schools. As a little guy, he was taught that when he said his prayers every night before bed, he should also pray that his true vocation be revealed to him. Every night, little Jimmy knelt beside his bed to pray, and along with blessing his family and friends, he requested his true vocation. One night when he was still in elementary school, he got up into his bed and his head had no sooner hit the pillow than he heard a distinctly female voice say, "How would you like to be a teacher?" He shot straight up in his bed, eyes wide with excitement and said, "Yeah – that's what I'm going to be. A teacher!"

When he first told me about this, I asked, "You actually got a voice that told you?" He looked puzzled. He asked, "What? Didn't you?" At the time he first told me about this, he was 56 years old and believed everyone got "the voice." I assured him that no, not everyone is so fortunate. Good thing he didn't know this when he got the voice, because he went right back to sleep with the certain knowledge that no matter what he did or studied, he was destined to teach. He taught middle school in the south Bronx, Fort Apache, for over 30 years. Many teachers pale at the thought of teaching there. He adored it. He was even made the Dean of Discipline. When asked about teaching in such a rough area, he would always say, "We had a great school. I never had to take a gun away from a kid. There was no trouble whatsoever. They knew what was expected of them."

I didn't meet Jim until after he had retired, but I learned from former students we had chance meetings with in the Bronx that they adored him as much as he adored teaching them. He cried after encountering former students – every time. They had beautiful families, amazing jobs (a policeman, a restaurant owner – it gives me goosebumps just to share this). These were kids that came from less than nothing. All because he got the voice.

Why am I telling you all this? Do you believe he really heard a voice as a kid? I do. I got the voice. I was 61 years old, a grieving widow wondering why she was hating her job. The voice was right between my eyes and clearly said, "It is time to just do what it is you've been so good at. For the rest of your life, you need to share with others all that you've learned and experienced. You need to be a life coach." I was stunned. It was the voice. What the voice said was perfect. Just like little Jimmy, I immediately felt with certainty that this is exactly what would happen. Nine months after Jim died, I walked into The Life Coach School and changed my world forever.

Learning to coach taught me more about myself than I thought possible. I mean, I thought I knew me – right? We all do. But there is so much more potential sitting inside of you than you can possibly realize. Once you begin to tap into just a little piece of that, life gets exciting. My certification was a double certification as a life coach and as a weight-loss coach. I am passionate about weight-loss coaching and that is the direction in which I took my life coaching practice. Initially, finding clients and spreading word about my approach to weight loss, which focused more on what drives us to overeat than on the actual foods, calories, and diet thinking, was going slow. I began working on launching a podcast called "Weight Coach" to help get my message out into the world. But as I was getting that podcast ready, there was a memory burning in my heart. As a new widow, I had gone into iTunes and searched for a podcast about being widowed. I just wanted to hear someone else's story and how they were dealing with the journey of widowhood. There was nothing. I was so shocked. I knew if I searched "Game of Thrones," there would be a hundred podcasts for that show. If I searched entrepreneurs, there would be hundreds. But there was not one podcast for widows.

It still lurked in the back of my mind – a constant nagging that there was nothing out there for widows in the form of podcast. I decided "Weight Coach" would have to wait just a little longer to be launched. I turned on my microphone, stared into the little recording meter ticking away on my computer screen and began to share my story. "Widow Cast" was born. Within less than 24 hours, I had finished sound editing on the first episode, acquired the artwork created for the podcast cover, purchased a hosting service for the recordings, and figured out how to get each recording to upload to iTunes, Google Play Music, and Stitcher (all apps to listen to podcasts). The podcast that I created straight from my heart for widows took on a life of its own.

On the podcast, I not only shared my story, but also incorporated a lot of information about the coaching tools I learned and used as a life coach because they had made such an impact on my own journey of widowhood. Listeners began to reach out to me in emails, seeking life coaching. The first session with the first widow that I agreed to coach was amazing. I was so elated at how much my coaching skills could help her, even after just the first session. Life coaching was powerful in helping the new widow grasp what she is experiencing and immediately begin to look toward her future. Not that she was bypassing her grief process, but she could embrace her process and know how to begin living again herself. My personal, emotional rewards from working with the women I have been blessed to coach are immense. To this day, I still feel so uplifted when I see the light come into someone's eyes.

So many widows were coming to me after having tried other professionals. I was being told things like, "I've paid a therapist for over two years and I still do not feel any better at all." "I started going to a grief counselor, but just couldn't go back after the second session. She was just off base. I didn't connect." "I tried a grief group, but had to stop because I was always even more depressed when I left a meeting than when I started."

I always asked the same question, "Was your therapist/counselor/psychologist a widow?" The inevitable answer was always, "No."

There is no degree in psychology that makes you understand what this is – widow grief. It is such a different experience from any other kind of loss. I lost my dad when I was in my late thirties, then lost my mom in my forties. I've lost close friends. This is entirely different. I study psychology. The truth is if someone asked me before Jim died, "If Jim dies, are you going to be okay?" I would've said, "Oh yes. I've experienced grief before. We've even talked about death between us. We have solid belief about the afterlife. I'll do fine." Not true. It was not anything like what I expected. In my mind, as I write this, I can see you, dear reader, nodding your head in solemn agreement. As widows, we know. Only another widow can truly get it. The realization finally dawned on me that there is so little available for widows. We need professionals who are also widows to work with other widows. We need widow coaches.

Chapter 2 – Me, a Widow Coach?

Are you ready to listen to "the voice"? Have others already been sending new widows in your direction, thinking you would be perfect to help them? Throughout your life, perhaps you've been the one that everyone comes to or opens up to. Like me, you may have already been coaching your coworkers in your role at work. Another contributing thought for me was the fact that I have always believed we create our own reality with our beliefs, expectations, and emotions. When I first saw the "thought model" when I was studying to be a life coach, it clicked immediately for me. "Whoa," I thought, "that is the exact formula for what I've always known to be true!" The Life Coach School taught me the single most powerful tool I have ever applied in my life. I danced all around this knowledge, and a lot of what Jim and I shared was our work at consciously creating our reality together for over 20 years. But when I saw how Brooke Castillo laid it out with such simplicity and in such a useable formula, it rocked my world. The concept that your thoughts are what create every feeling you ever have, and those feelings cause you to act or not take any action at all, which produces the results in your life was not new to me. But seeing it in a formula was. In a very basic description, it looks like this:

C: (circumstance in your life – this is the bare facts)
T: (your thought – it is the sentence that plays in your brain in response to the facts above)
F: (the feeling your thought produces – it is one word)
A: (the actions you take or don't take because of the feeling)
R: (the result your actions create in your life)

So again, the interpretation of this is the circumstances in your life are bare facts, without judgment. This is the part you have no control over. Your thoughts are what you tell yourself about the facts in your reality. Those thoughts create your feelings. How you act or don't act is a result of how you are feeling (or how you do not want to feel). The results you create in your life are created by your actions. It all starts on that "T" line with your thought!

As you read through this book, we will revisit the concepts presented in the thought model. Much of what you read in this book may change how you think about things forever. Would it be worth certifying as a widow coach to work with others? I can tell you with no reservation that reaching out and helping widows has given me the greatest reward of my life. My entire career is now based on doing something that makes a difference in the world. Every day I wake up looking forward to my work and loving what I get to do. This profession not only helped me get through my own journey of widowhood, it has changed the entire trajectory of my life. Widow coaches coaching other widows is the perfect system of healing and recovery. Working in class and learning beside other widows can inspire you and create clarity around what you now want in your life.

Some of the widows in my class indeed go on to become widow coaches. But others uncover a dream they had long forgotten and then integrate it with what they've learned as a widow coach. Some want to create a healing center that offers yoga, meditation, massage, and coaching in a nurturing environment for widows. One widow had a long-time dream of opening a bed and breakfast by the ocean, but came to see how effective and rewarding it would be to host a B&B for widows so they could get out of their daily environment into a space of comfort and renewal at a place exclusive to widows and widowers. Another widow coach is in the process of establishing a legacy foundation. I stand in awe of these women who come to my class and then create dreams that blow my mind!

This is where you begin to feel alive again after months, even years of just going through a daily existence to survive. Even if you do not think you would go forward as a certified widow coach to set up a practice to coach others, learning the tools and applying them is true evolution toward the best of who you are. This is where you step out of the flames and ashes of finding yourself widowed into the light of your own path. Welcome, widow coach.

Chapter 3 – It's Not Enough to Be an Empathic Friend

I was interviewing a widow who was interested in becoming a certified widow coach in my class. She said she had made tremendous strides and wanted to pay it forward. She went on to tell me how so many other widows have crossed her path in the last couple of years, and she would help by sharing her story. I told her how wonderful this was because just sharing your story with a new widow can indeed be helpful to her. But then she went on to tell me about all the "advice" she was giving, and how empathic she was. She would always cry because in her eyes, this was offering consolation to them. I gently tried to explain that if she was crying, then the new widow could not freely open up about her own tears. That this was being a wonderful girlfriend to the widow, but it was not coaching.

I tried to explain to her about "holding space" for another human so they could feel safe and supported in their own pain without having to accommodate her pain too. She just couldn't get it unfortunately. Apparently she thought I was some kind of unemotional monster. Lord, I'm a widow! It's not possible to be unemotional. I was trying to gently explain that dumping out all her own pain on the new widow was not helpful. Well, I take that back. It was helpful in a way if it was cathartic for her. But it was not helping the other widow. We both agreed she was not a good fit for Widow Coaches Class because there was a fundamental difference in our definition of what it means to help another.

"Holding space" means that we are willing to walk alongside another person in whatever journey they're on without judging them, making them feel inadequate, trying to fix them, or trying to impact the outcome. When we hold space for other people, we open our hearts, offer unconditional support, and let go of judgment and control. Widows need to know that there are some people with whom they can be vulnerable and weak without fear of being judged.

Holding space for another is the greatest gift you can offer to someone drowning in emotional pain. It means that you are able to listen to them not only without judgement, but also without expectation. You do not agree or disagree. You do not react. You stay neutral. Why is this so very important? You are allowing them to unload their mind and in return, receive an honest perspective. This is often the most difficult part of coaching because it requires you to coach yourself first. It requires that you listen to your client and hear what they are saying without making any immediate assumptions about it. What they are telling you is not about you. The minute you start to identify with it, you make it about you instead of about them.

We have a very human tendency to want to fix people, give them advice, or judge them for not being further along the path than they are, but we must hold space because we know that it's important. At the same time, you need people in your life that you can trust to hold space for you.

This is one of the reasons a large part of my teaching for my widow coaches is how to coach themselves. Unless you can coach yourself and arrive at a place of having no expectations from your client, you cannot be an effective coach. You have to learn that it is not your job to try and offer an immediate "feel better" approach. That's like slapping a Band-Aid on a broken leg. If you truly want to help and allow the widow to walk away with a new perspective, it is going to sometimes mean that she is not immediately feeling wonderful. But she has been able to tell you her deepest thoughts without worry of being ashamed. She will have been given a new perspective on her thinking that is going to make a huge difference to her.

To truly support people in their own growth, transformation, grief, etc., we can't do it by taking their power away (trying to fix their problems), shaming them (implying that they should know more than they do), or overwhelming them (giving them more information than they're ready for). We have to be prepared to step to the side so that they can make their own choices, offer them unconditional love and support, give gentle guidance when it's needed, and make them feel safe even when they make mistakes. When you do not assume that you know what is best for your client and instead allow them to find their own inner wisdom, you may be surprised at what YOU can learn FROM your client. Allow them to make different decisions and to have different experiences than you would.

A client who was not a widow came to me about weight loss. In the process of working with her, I began to learn that a lot of her emotional overeating was because she was sure her husband was cheating on her. This is actually not an uncommon theme in weight-loss coaching. When a woman feels unloved or unlovable, she will often turn to food for the comfort she no longer feels with her spouse. But as I listened to her story more and more, my mind was saying, "Oh, my gosh, he is absolutely cheating on her." Everything pointed to it in her story. I was being completely drawn in by her story and began believing it was true. Not once did I verbalize that, however, and I would coach myself on the topic an hour before every session with her so I could remain neutral. It was necessary not to immediately believe her side of the story. By coaching myself, I could see that I was only hearing one side of this without any provable facts. I could more clearly understand that what I was hearing was my client's thoughts, and that is where the true work was needed. In coaching, we could not change her husband, but we could change her thoughts about herself.

Even with the best of intentions, it is human to judge your clients, both in positive and in negative ways. When we are coaching widow-to-widow, we are going to naturally empathize with most of what they are saying and feeling. It is natural to compare the widow's story to our own and make judgments.

But you must realize your own judgment will only interfere with your ability to help your client. Coaching yourself on your thoughts about your client's story will allow you to acknowledge your own opinion about it and let it go.

If I had not been able to hold space for my weight-loss client, if I had agreed with her that he was absolutely cheating on her, I would have never been able to help her heal the pain around this issue. As we worked through her pain and her thoughts, guess what happened? The realization dawned that she was not certain he was cheating. As we worked through more and more of her thoughts and emotions, it became clear how her belief he was cheating was clouding her interpretation of every event. As we got closer and closer to the facts of her life, there was no true evidence he was doing anything wrong. There was certainly evidence that he loved her and was there to be with her. I learned a huge lesson with that client. It was proof that holding the space for her, particularly by not buying into her story with her, was what truly made a difference in the end. The truth was, it did not matter if he was cheating or was not cheating. What mattered was what my client made it mean about her. What mattered most was the emotional pain my client was experiencing. That is what needed fixing.

As a certified widow coach, you will be so much more than a "good friend" to the widows you are helping. You will be a facilitator, coach, and guide. With gentle, nonjudgmental guidance and insight, you are going to help each widow you work with walk one of the most difficult journeys of her life.

You are going to walk alongside her without judging her, making her feel inadequate, or trying to fix her because you think you know the best outcome for her. You don't – only she can discover this. When you hold space, you truly open your heart to another and let go of control over the outcome.

When you overly identify with the story a client is telling you, you are getting right into the pool of water with her. She is drowning in her emotional pain. If you jump right in to save a drowning human, they will grab onto you and both of you will go down together. In other words, not only have you not helped them, you've so identified with them that you've just drowned as well. Instead, if you can stay out of their pool (their story), now you are capable of tossing a life preserver from the shore. So stay conscious in a coaching session and become aware if you are beginning to slip right into the pool with your client.

Keep your own ego out of it! When you think you know what they should be doing or feeling, you are taking away their power. You are making that widow feel even more useless and powerless than she felt when she came to you for help in the first place. I know we want to make them better right away. We want to say, just do this, just think this. But it is far better to show her how to look at her own thoughts and ideas. It empowers her if she can, with your gentle guidance and support, see her own thinking and find her own solutions. Your client may surprise you. You may learn something from her!

Widows often have thoughts that they cannot bear to think. It is only when you create an open space for her where she feels safe and that it is okay to be completely herself that she will be able to openly admit to herself some of the thoughts she is having. Maybe she is secretly extremely hurt by something she came across in her husband's things after he passed away. She has not told another soul. She has not even completely admitted to herself that she is thinking about it. But it is being held deep inside and creating such pain for her. If you show up with tenderness, strength, compassion, and a mind free of judgment, she is going to be able to share that discovery and thought with you and free herself of this dark, painful secret.

Give your clients a space that is safe enough for them to fall apart in. They need a space where they can fall in before they can get back up again. Allow them to make decisions that are not what you would have "recommended." Their decision may lead them to a powerful place that you could not have foreseen.

The widow I interviewed for widow coach certification was completely unwilling to acknowledge that there may be more she could do for the widows she so wanted to help. She was convinced that agreeing with their pain and breaking down and crying were more compassionate than being open and supportive to provide space for them. Her heart was completely in the right place, but she was not open to learning something more. She just wanted to be right. When you insist on being right, you are pressuring the person you are helping to conform to your thoughts and emotions instead of teaching them to explore their own.

Holding space is not something that can be mastered overnight or just by reading my descriptions above. It is something you have to practice and become acutely aware of. This only happens through knowing how to coach yourself about your own preconceived notions and ideas. Learning how to hold space and developing the skill will reward you not only in your ability as a coach, but in your ability to support the people around you in your daily life. You will better understand how to "be there" for a friend in need.

Chapter 4 – The Stories We Repeat

There was a fantastic news story about a little girl in England that pulled a sword out of the lake believed to be the lake that holds King Arthur's sword. How fantastic is *that*! King Arthur received Excalibur from The Lady of the Lake at Dozmary Pool and when he was dying, he returned and threw Excalibur back into Dozmary. Along comes a little girl 16 centuries later and pulls a sword out of the lake. I mean, come ON.

When she first told her dad she could see a sword under the water, he said, "Don't be silly, it is probably just a piece of fencing." But no, she pulled Excalibur out of the shallow water. Her dad says he believes it is most likely a movie prop left behind. He says that the sword appears to be only 20 to 30 years old. I am executing my very best seven-year-old eye roll – dads are like that. My dad was like that. If I had pulled a one-pound diamond out of the earth, he would've said, "It's probably just glass, Jo Jo. Put it back."

What I want to hear is *her* story about this sword - before she starts believing what her "Da" says. I bet it is a wonderful story about swimming in Dozmary, perhaps secretly pretending The Lady of the Lake was there when she first spotted the hilt underwater. "Da" didn't believe her, but she believed and reached out to take the sword from The Lady of the Lake. A much better story than "bits of fencing" or old movie props! I hope she spins this for all it's worth and enjoys every second of holding Excalibur in her keeping.

Remember the coaching model I showed you in Chapter 2? Let's break down the difference between the circumstances and the thoughts. The actual facts of what happened, is what both of them would agree on:

They were paddling around Dozmary Pool.

She spotted something metal underwater.

She pulled a sword out of Dozmary.

Those are the facts of reality. Anything more is story and belief. Her dad's story is no more plausible than what her story of the sword may be, or even what my presumed story for her might be! I think *my* story is far more fun to believe and could even lead the trajectory of this little girl's future. She might become more of a risk taker, believing firmly in herself, for she clearly knows a sword from a bit of fencing, eh?

This, my friends, is exactly how we create our lives. It is not so much about the facts of reality as it is what we believe about them. There are all kinds of possible stories to spin around the facts – stories that make us feel insignificant or stories that can make us feel like we could wield Excalibur in the world. The story we choose to believe will 100% affect the destiny we play out in the world.

We all have our story about the loss of our spouse. I remember when my father passed away, my mom would tell everyone about it. I mean *everyone*. The mailman, her nail lady, and every grocery checker she would encounter heard the whole emotionally upsetting story of my dad's illness and death. They would be treated to hearing how encountering some of the oxygen tubing in the bottom of the clothing hamper a week after he died made her break down all over again. She was not telling this to us or to a counselor. She kept recounting it over and over again to perfect strangers. At first, I was embarrassed by it. Then I figured, she needed to retell this story repeatedly to "get it out of her system." It never got out of her system. She did not let it go for years. It kept her trapped in her pain.

It was not the retelling that created so much pain for her. It was the story she had created around my dad's death that kept her reliving such pain. There were options for a better story. He had been diagnosed with asbestosis, a fancy word that means he contracted cancer of the esophagus from the repeated exposure to asbestos while working in underground Nike missile sites as part of his career in the Army. He was in the advanced stages, meaning it was metastasizing to his other organs and primarily to his brain. Dad was a highly intelligent man. Seeing his brain begin to fail was indeed heartbreaking. Finally hospitalized, he was struggling with the last days of the disease. He was kept mostly comfortable. He died on Father's Day with all of us there around him and "Happy Father's Day" cards all taped up around his bed. Dad was released from the struggle. He would still be "Dad" in the hereafter.

That was my story. It still hurt to lose him. Yes, I cried a lot over the ensuing weeks. But I healed. I held a story made up of mostly facts and some positive thoughts about his death. This was a very big difference from what I could have been telling myself about the loss of my dad.

The first thing you need to know is there is your 'story' versus the actual facts of the event. Facts are neutral. They do not including feelings and judgments. Facts are just facts. You can prove facts in a court of law beyond a doubt. Everyone would agree with the facts. All the rest is your story and what you chose to tell yourself about the facts. The facts in my story: Dad worked in Nike missile sites while in the Army. There was asbestos in those sites. The doctors diagnosed him with esophageal cancer that was caused by asbestos exposure. The cancer had metastasized. He died in the hospital on Father's Day.

These are facts. Parts of my story like, "Dad was a highly intelligent man. Seeing his brain begin to fail was indeed heartbreaking. Finally hospitalized, he was struggling in the last days of the disease. He was kept mostly comfortable," are all my thoughts about it. These are thoughts, not facts, because they are judgments. I cannot prove he was kept comfortable. He was not awake to tell us he was okay and without pain. I cannot prove he was struggling in the last days. This is my own assessment. Someone else may have seen it very differently. Even the thought that my dad was highly intelligent could be subjective. Someone else may have had an encounter with my dad and walked away thinking, "What an idiot!"

You might notice that most of the thoughts in my story about my dad's death are very comforting thoughts. I could choose very distressful thoughts like "Father's Day is always going to be hurtful and hard to face." The only purpose that thought would serve is to make me feel awful every year on Father's Day. Do you see that? Instead I can choose to think, "I will always remember my dad on Father's Day."

Write down your story – the one you tell about the death of your husband. Write it down in detail. Then as you read it back, begin to notice what the facts are. What everyone would agree with. The facts may look something like this:

My husband was ill.

My husband died.

He died at home.

Those would be the facts. All the rest would be the story you tell about it; all your thoughts about it. So begin to look at those sentences that include adjectives and judgment. Ask yourself how each sentence feels when you think it. Is it uncomfortable? Is it hurtful? Do you begin to see how the thoughts you choose (and thoughts are all optional) create the painful emotions you feel?

Another example is a widow who came to me for coaching about a month after her husband died. One of her concerns was that she took quite a bit of time away from work when he was ill in the hospital to be by his side. Then after his death, she continued to take time off. It had been about six weeks all totaled that she had been off of work at the time of our first call together. Her thought was that her coworkers were thinking that she just needed to get it together and return to her job. This was very distressing for her because she truly did not feel ready to go back to work yet. It had only been four weeks since he died. Then I inquired what her job was. She was the manager of the emergency room in a major hospital. No surprise that she was distressed over the thought of returning to her job too soon. We talked in depth about what her coworkers were thinking and how they might have been pressuring her to return to work.

The facts are these:

She took two weeks off to be by her dying husband's side.

He died.

She had not returned to work yet.

Everything else was story. Total story! The truth was that she had not talked to any of her coworkers. She had been avoiding talking to anyone at the hospital because she was feeling ashamed that she was still not back at work. She was thinking *they* were thinking she should be "over it" and back at work. But no one said that. She had no way of knowing for sure that this is what they were thinking. When we explored it further, she realized they were probably thinking the exact opposite. It was in exploring her entire story that we were finally able to identify the facts and then discuss everything else that was left.

If you are dwelling on stories from your past, it is time to start looking at them as you think about today. The truth is that the only things that can affect you in this very moment are the thoughts you are having about the past.

It is not useful to explain your current condition based on something that happened to you in your past. We will often point to incidents that happened to us as children as why we are feeling like we do today. But the incidents of our childhood no longer exist anywhere but in our minds. Have you ever talked to a sibling about something you both witnessed as children and been shocked to hear your sibling describe it completely differently? That is just how malleable the past is, according to our thoughts and interpretation of it. That is fabulous news. It means you can look to something in your past that still upsets you, write out your story, and separate the facts from your thoughts. Once you do that, you can see what parts of your story have been optional. You will see what parts of the story have been hurting you over and over again over the years. Once you realize that you can't even be sure that most of those thoughts are true, then you can start having other thoughts about it. You can choose thoughts in your present that are more supportive.

Your past is the story you tell about it. Change the story, and you literally change your past.

Chapter 5 – What Do You Believe?

One of the most shocking parts of losing your spouse is also losing your own sense of identity. It is as if our ego, our very persona, is shattered on rocks and all the shards are scattered in front of us. That question of, "Who am I now?" is asked by many, many widows. Who you are now all comes down to what you believe about yourself and your life. You held beliefs that were very different before your spouse died. You believed the two of you would walk into the sunset of life together, hand in hand. You did not believe for one minute that you would be walking that path on your own.

In the last chapter, you learned about the difference between story and fact. Whenever someone tells you about their life and their experiences, they will give you a handful of actual facts with a whole lot of story and thoughts. Every one of us takes what happens to us and decides what it means in our life. We create the "story" of who we are and what our lives are about. Many choose to look back at the challenges and trials of widowhood and believe they are unlucky in life, or that having it be constant pain and struggle is just how it is supposed to be. There are people who think they are just no good because of situations they had been involved in or things that happened to them.

We can choose to believe we are our circumstances. We can choose to believe we are defined by our loss. We can choose to believe we are the mistakes we've made in our past and that we are doomed to make the same mistakes over and over. We can choose to believe we are doomed, period!

It is not the events in our lives that shape who we are; it is what we chose to believe about those events. It is about what we choose to make the events mean to us and about us. Rarely have most of us consciously made those choices! If we could consciously choose, we might want to choose to think we have a big, wonderful life. But that thought is a steep step for a widow or widower to mentally embrace. A big, wonderful life can happen, but it is going to take a lot of small steps to rebuild our belief in ourselves.

Much depends on how the widow interprets her life through the lens of her loss. The experience itself does not shape her present and her future, but what she makes her loss mean does. The grief continues, yes it does. But much of the emotional pain of the widow's present is based around her beliefs about being widowed.

There are widows who interpret their life without their spouse to be exactly what was modeled for them in the past by widowed friends or widowed relatives. Perhaps those widows played out huge dramas and told everyone who would listen that their lives were now worthless. So the new widow believes her life is truly over and acts as she believes she is expected to.

As widows, we can have many illogical beliefs surrounding our thoughts. One of my immediate beliefs after my husband died was that I would become a bag lady. I would end up with only a shopping cart of belongings, living under some underpass. Even though I knew full well how our beliefs can shape our actual reality and that this thought was going to be very detrimental to my own future, it was difficult to coach myself through that thought. If you believe you are always going to be strapped for money, then that is just what you will create and experience in your life. If your reality is not immediately reflecting that belief, it is going to set up a tension in your life because your world and your belief about it do not match up. When your beliefs about your life and your actual reality do not match up, either your life will shift to match your belief or your belief needs to shift. I decided my belief about becoming a bag lady had to shift, and quickly! If I did not work on my beliefs that surrounded my ability to take care of my own finances, I would end up sabotaging my own budget or passing up opportunities to make an income. I would, in fact, create becoming financially insolvent.

Have you thought that you are now destined to live your life alone, in a lonely space? Can you look at that thought and see that it might be illogical? Are you going to be completely alone for every second of every day for the rest of your life? Start to become aware of your thoughts and your beliefs.

Learn to question them. As a widow coach, you learn how to help your clients see and understand how their thoughts and beliefs are creating the results they are seeing in their lives. Do you wonder what you believe? Look around you. What is in your life right now? What *is* your life right now? That is exactly what you have believed. Your present life is a pure reflection of what you have believed and expected. Many of us need to begin to nurture a belief that we deserve something more – just like we need to help our clients write out their stories and identify the facts versus their thoughts and beliefs. We also need to help them understand how these play out in their lives to create their reality.

As a coach, it is critical that you do this work for yourself first. You need to be walking down the path, just ahead of your clients, so that you can lead the way out of despair.

Chapter 6 – Basic Emotional Needs

Tony Robbins, early in his carrier, identified six core human needs. These needs play a powerful role in his coaching. When I began coaching widows, I found this concept amazing for helping a widow identify what is import in her life going forward; and how to make sure it is being fulfilled. These needs are identified as:

- Certainty
- Variety
- Significance
- Love & connection
- Growth
- Contribution

Certainty and variety are opposites that pair together to create a balance in life. Significance pairs with love and connection. If one is tilted too far, our need the other will become more of a priority. The last pair, growth and contribution, are needs of the spirit and one complements the other. We experience all six of these needs. But the difference for each of us is in which we prioritize.

Which needs are our top priority in life? When a widow experiences the loss of her spouse, she suddenly feels as if there are gaping holes in her soul. Her life is empty in more ways than one. Those holes in her soul are needs that her spouse was fulfilling for her. Now she struggles because these emotional needs are no longer being met in any way.

Do we need another person to fulfill our needs? Absolutely not. We want to be able to feel fulfilled as an individual. This is true whether we are alone or in a relationship. It is in our psyche to fulfill our priority needs. So much so that we will unconsciously fulfill those needs in a positive way or a destructive way. That's right. We will fall into ways of meeting an emotional need that are self-destructive in our desperation to fill that void in our emotional life. This is why it is so important to review your client's priorities and help her decide, consciously, exactly how she wants to fulfill her priorities. So let's take a closer look at each of these.

Certainty

This is our need to feel in control and know what is coming next so we can feel secure. It is comfort in planning ahead, or in having a "method" that we follow. It is a survival mechanism that wants to make sure we are safe and stable. A high need for certainty does not want to take risks in life. Often a widow finds herself in an unstable financial situation when her spouse dies and this elevates a sudden increase in the need to feel certainty.

Variety

This is *uncertainty*. Those with a high need for variety are the risk takers, the explorers. Those with a need for variety travel more. They love adventure sports. Variety is a way to feel engaged and alive. If you spend all your energy in a place of certainty/comfort/security, eventually you begin to feel stagnant and yearn for something out of the box. The need for variety kicks in!

Significance

We all want to feel special and unique in the world. There is a good chance that your spouse was the one who made you feel this way on a regular basis. This is how we distinguish ourselves from others, or sometimes even above others. One can gain a feeling of significance by achieving success with a degree or a business success. Sometimes spending money can make you feel significant. Go out and indulge in something and you come home feeling pretty good about yourself. Of course, missing out on being significant in our spouse's life can lead to disastrous spending sprees in an unconscious effort to fill that void! You will start to see the positive ways to fulfill an emotional need as well as negative ways.

Love & Connection

This is the breath of our life. We all crave love and connection as human beings. When we are in love, we feel fully alive. When we lose love, the pain is unbearable. We can nurture love and connection in our life through friends, prayer, family, even walking in nature. Initially, widows want to pull in family close and this happens for us around the funeral. But as time goes by, our family has their own lives. It is no secret that friends drop away after widowhood. Widows find they are isolated and alone. You need to build new friendships in life. Connecting with other widows can create very strong bonds.

The four needs listed above are all needs of the personality and work like opposing forces in our lives. For example, if our need for significance is a very high priority in our life and we do not feel it is being met, we will sacrifice nurturing any love and connection to put all our focus and energy into creating our significance in the world. Have you ever met the professional who is so focused on their work they ignore their family?

If you create so much certainty in your life because you have a high need for certainty, eventually you begin to feel a little bored with the sameness of it all. You begin to yearn to travel or some other way to shake up your life a little. You yearn for a little variety! We will absolutely find ways to fulfill these needs; whether it be achieving a new profession or constantly playing the "one-upmanship game" to make us feel more significant than the next person. The next two needs below are spiritual needs. Not all people ever fulfill these needs. If you do take steps to fulfill these next two needs, you will feel truly fulfilled.

Growth

This is the need to expand your own capabilities and learning. It is taking on new things and stretching to reach your full potential, becoming a better version of you. If you are not growing, you are dying. Our spouse dies and we just stop in place. Our very soul begins to atrophy because we've stopped striving for something more.

Contribution

This is a sense of being of service to others. It is the need to share who we are with others. If something incredible happens in your life, your first instinct is to call someone to share it with. We want to give to others. It is our nature. Helping and supporting others is what gives life meaning.

One of my favorite examples of Certainty versus Variety is reality TV stars Chip and Joanna Gaines of *Fixer Upper* on HGTV. If you've followed this show from the beginning, you have seen how they strongly demonstrate these two characteristics. Chip is all about variety. He loves risk, the element of surprise! Joanna is all about certainty. She likes things planned out well and put into motion in a safe, consistent manner. Joanna does *not* appreciate the element of surprise. Yet the relationship between the two of them is perfect. They clearly see that the other has an element that balances them out. Chip brings Joanna to the forefront of life. Joanna grounds Chip in life. If you want to see what this means, check out *I Am Second's* "White Chair Film" of Chip and Joanna Gaines. This video interview is one of the best examples of the contrast, and I always ask my students to watch it. Then we consider what we would need to coach Joanna on if she were suddenly without Chip, and what would we coach Chip on if Joanna were gone.

When her emotional needs are suddenly no longer being met due to the death of a spouse, a widow might feel she has no control over the situation in which she finds herself. She is at risk of giving up and engaging in addictive and/or destructive behaviors as a way of creating comfort in her life. My own *modus operandi* in life has been emotional eating. I had worked through this, however, and had dropped most of my excess weight. Moreover, it was staying completely off because I had coached and understood what urged me to overeat in the past. Yet six weeks after Jim suddenly died, I realized I had put on 20 pounds! I fell right back into a destructive behavior pattern in an effort to provide comfort to myself. As soon as I realized this, I was able to look for other avenues to meet my emotional needs.

Many widows who have come to me for coaching turned to alcohol and overdrinking. One widow I worked with had hit rock bottom with drinking and was able to get that under control, only to begin overeating and gaining weight. She was trading one compensation for another. Eating, drinking, worrying, smoking, or other undesirable behaviors can be a quick and direct way for us to get out of pain and into pleasure. But the pleasure of that is fleeting, and we are left with addiction. If you think, do, or feel something that meets multiple emotional needs, you will become addicted to the behavior. Going out in the evening to drink can create variety in your life. It also feels like it helps you connect to others who are there drinking, fulfilling a bit of your need for love and connection. It becomes your routine to do this and you can count on it to relax you and count on your drinking buddies to also be there. That makes it feel secure and provides certainty. Is there any wonder that it would be extremely difficult to give that up? These can be difficult patterns to break out of. But it is not impossible if we can be shown why we are being destructive and understand what it is we are trying to provide in our life.

When you are exploring your client's priorities, speaking in terms of the six needs listed above will not make sense to her. But if you prompt her to think about what is important in her life right now, she will come up with things like her kids, her job, wanting to travel more, or self-care, among many other possibilities. You want to help her create a list of the priorities in her life, and walk her through comparing one to the other to determine which feels more critical, more urgent. Then help her explore exactly what she can do to make sure she is fulfilling the top two or three needs that are most important to her in life.

Chapter 7 – Moving Past the Pain

There is a great little app that I downloaded onto my iPad called TimeHop. It will show me posts I made on Facebook or Twitter from the same date over the last eight years or so. It also pulls up any photos I had taken on that day in the past. A few days ago, I opened up TimeHop, and one of the things that came up from four years ago was a short bit of video showing two plates on a diner table with hamburgers on them. Clearly I was fiddling with my cell phone camera and accidentally had it on video instead of snapping a picture. As soon as I saw those hamburgers, I knew exactly what it was. It was Hamburger Tuesday. I shared the "throwback memory" on Facebook and said, "I miss our Hamburger Tuesdays. This was Jim's favorite part of the week." Another widow commented on the memory saying she found it so disconcerting how we could be overwhelmed by a memory, a smell, or a taste. I know that we've all experienced those moments as widows. A random song on the radio while you are driving home from running errands, and suddenly you are sobbing over your steering wheel.

A sweet reminder does not have to overwhelm us with depression and sadness. It all depends on where your head is when the memory hits you. I was just randomly flipping through the posts in my TimeHop app on my phone when this bit of video from four years ago came up. My first thought was how much I miss our Hamburger Tuesdays. Our local diner has a special menu of gourmet hamburgers for just $5 on Tuesdays. Jim loved a good burger, and loved a bargain even more. So we instituted Hamburger Tuesdays as a regular tradition.

I could have wailed and told myself I will never have another Hamburger Tuesday with my sweetheart again. I could have been devastated and told all my friends how this just "came out of nowhere and now my heart is breaking all over again." I could have chosen to spend my Sunday in deep depression and yet again re-experience the crushing pain of losing my best friend, my partner in hamburglar crime, my sweetheart. But I didn't do any of that.

It was a deep tug on my heart. But before it could spiral into deep pain, I chose to shift my thoughts and thus shift my emotions. I remembered how it was not so much about the burgers, but about the two of us giggling like kids because it felt like it was such a steal to get gourmet burgers for $5. It was also our special time together, laughing over the cheapest date night on earth.

I could smile to myself over our $5 date nights and how we would take that time to really re-connect with each other. It was amazing how after 20 years we would sit down to burgers in a diner and still laugh and chat together like young lovers.

That tug on the heart turned into sweet remembrance. All because I have learned how to manage my thoughts and feel my emotions without any resistance. I chose to tell myself (and others) a different story of this bit of video from four years ago.

I did not always have this skill. It is not something that is ingrained in most of us. As I mentioned before, I had struggled with my weight for decades because of emotional eating. Emotions were overwhelming to me. I was afraid of feeling them, so I learned at a young age that if I was eating, I was not even noticing my feelings. I could dull out the feelings with food. When Jim first died, I thought I was handling it well; considering how sudden it was and my inability to focus on anything initially. But when I finally realized that my morning routine had been completely out of whack since his death and there were days that I did not even remember to brush my teeth, I wrote down all my morning steps on a 3x5 card so I could again ingrain those simple morning routine things. One of those steps was to weigh myself. When I saw that 20-pound gain on the scale, I immediately knew I had not been "handling it" as well as I thought I had been. Clearly, there had been emotional eating. It was my way of trying to buffer out the deep emotional pain because I was fearful of feeling the full weight of my sadness.

Buffering happens in many ways. Overeating is just one of them. Every one of the widows who came to me for coaching because of their drinking after their husbands died told me she had never had any kind of drinking issue in the past. Yet in the lingering pain over the death of their husband, they turned to alcohol and could not control it. I have not one iota of judgment about that. I know it is the same mechanism that caused me to overeat. It is the same mechanism that can cause someone to overspend money, or gamble, or spend hours and hours on social media. Buffering can also be keeping yourself "too busy" to do anything, especially too busy to even think about your life and the deep pain waiting just under your emotional surface. It is the fear and discomfort of the pain that causes those buffering behaviors. We think if we feel that overwhelming emotional pain, it will never stop.

The truth about feelings is they only last about 90 seconds if we are willing to allow them. Oh, they can return, just like waves on the beach. However, each time the feeling is a little less intense. The feelings are only overwhelming when we resist feeling the emotion, or we continue to spin a story about how terrible the feeling or event is. It is when we can allow the feeling and invite it in that we discover the feeling cannot kill us. The feeling is not going to last forever. You can even feel a feeling like deep sadness and then invite another feeling, like the sweet pleasure of remembrance I felt over seeing a video clip of our Hamburger Tuesday. It is important that we do feel our emotions fully. It is part of being human. Our thoughts create emotions in our body.

Where do you find your feeling? Take a second and notice an emotion you are feeling. Ask yourself where you feel it *in your body*. This is where feelings happen. Fear can feel like a sudden clenching in the stomach, or perhaps butterflies in the tummy. Depression and sadness makes my arms and legs feel like they are sandbags and I can barely lift them. If I'm especially blue, I can even feel it in my cheeks – like they are pulling downward. Depression is a cold, blue, downward feeling. That is how I describe it. When I stop and notice all this, the feeling begins to subside almost immediately. As soon as you start to ask yourself questions about your feeling, like what color it is, where it is in your body, if it is hot or cold or neither; then the feeling processes and eases up.

If you instead resist the feeling – you want to push it away with food, drink, smoking, whatever – it becomes stronger and stronger. It is like trying to hold a beach ball underwater with one hand. The harder you push it down, the harder you feel that ball pushing back up against your hand. Then, when you do let the ball go, it shoots up out of the water with force! Just like an emotion you cannot stuff down any longer. If you let that emotion just stay with you, like a beach ball just floating on the water next to you, it will drift away.

Ultimately, you can think about how you would like to feel instead. Rewrite your story like we did in chapter 4. Make it a good one. Inspire the feelings you would rather feel. I'm not saying you cannot choose to feel sadness. For sure we would choose to feel sad over the death of our spouse. You can choose that emotion and allow it completely. That is different than trying not to feel it. Allow your sadness. Describe it for yourself. Recognize it when sadness shows up. Our life as humans is going to include negative emotions. It is how we know when we feel the positive emotions. If you never, ever felt sad, how would you recognize when you felt happy? Part of our experience on this planet are emotions that are just going to feel yucky. But it is okay to feel them. We can handle it. Once you know that no feeling is going to last forever and that you are okay with feeling it, then there is nothing you cannot face. You can do anything. You can feel anything.

That is where tremendous growth enters into your life. When you know you can experience any emotion that comes your way and that it is not going to last forever, then you are willing to step out and try things you never imagined before. Fear? No problem. You knew when you applied for a new job it was going to feel scary. So welcome that fear on in and apply anyway. Grief? We know how we can chose to experience that, and even feel it as beautiful remembrance of the time we had together with our spouse. Now you begin to grow as a human being. Out of the pure trauma of losing someone you loved dearly, you can experience tremendous personal growth. It is not tarnishing your memories or the legacy of your husband's life. It is showing the world all the glory of your memories and the legacy of your husband's life. It is when you do not allow your feelings and let them process through your body that you keep yourself in a place of pain and struggle. The fact that you can choose to laugh again and be excited about something you are trying for the first time is a beautiful testimony to the love you shared. You get to feel everything, good and bad.

Chapter 8 – The Power of Asking the Right Questions

Knowing what questions to ask is key in finding the cause of your client's unhappiness. I coached a widow who came to me saying she could not get anything done. She just could not start things and if she did start something, she could not finish it. She said the fog of her loss was still so powerful she could not accomplish even the simplest tasks. She was completely mystified why she could not do anything, but knew she could not continue her life this way.

We could try to guess or assume we already know why she is feeling this way. Or we could tell her how we felt that way too and it is okay. But she is saying it is not okay anymore. It is complete hubris to assume you know why this widow is struggling with this because you can identify with how she is feeling. The only way you are going to know for sure what is causing this lack of focus for her is to ask questions. Lots of questions. They do not have to be complex. In fact, the most powerful question in my coaching toolbox is only three letters long: "Why?"

The best coaching does not advise someone on what they need to do based on what the coach thinks is best. The best coaching uncovers what is causing the client's emotions and creating the unwanted results in her life, and then helps her see that perspective so that she can discover what it is she truly needs to do. So when she says, "I cannot do anything or finish anything," you ask, "Why?" Then you *listen.* Then ask why again and listen.

By asking why, you can show her how she has created her current circumstances and/or perpetuated the emotional pain of loss by how she is choosing to think about it. It is critical that you help your client recognize what she has been thinking and feeling, and help her see that those thoughts and feelings have been affecting what she has been doing that is creating the results in her life. Widows will come to you and tell they are stuck in life because of things that happened to them or their circumstances in life. They truly have no idea what they want in their lives, or they do, but have a million reasons why they can't have it. They will blame their loss, the culture, their family, their job, their entire situation. Coaching shows your clients that they alone have created what they are experiencing in how they are thinking about it. Being stuck isn't something that happened *to them.* Being stuck is about the story they have been telling themselves. I can almost guarantee that this will not be something they want to hear at first, because it feels like they are being *blamed* for their feelings and their life. When they begin to see that it's not about blame, but about taking responsibility for what they think and how they feel, it can be very empowering. The fact that they created this, they actually chose this, means they can create something different. It is in their power to change it.

Here is the trick about asking questions. If you ask a negative question, you are going to get negative responses. It is what the brain does. It is a computer sitting between our ears! Just like programming a computer, "garbage in, garbage out." If you ask your client why she is so depressed, her brain will kick out all the reasons she has to be depressed. If you ask your client why she cannot do anything or complete anything, her brain will give a myriad of reasons why she cannot possibly accomplish anything. If instead you ask your client why she should be grateful right now, her brain will provide lots of reasons her life is good. She is going to feel completely differently in answering that question than she would feel if she was telling you all the reasons she has to be depressed! Ask her how she could get something completed. If she says, "I don't know," ask her if she did know, what would it be? The truth is, she does know. Our brain tries to shut down and be lazy by saying, "I don't know." It is easier than trying to come up with an answer. But we always have the answer.

We ask ourselves questions in our heads constantly. Try to eavesdrop on your mind to see what it is you ask yourself. Is it a negative question or a positive question? Can you change up your question so that it feels wonderful to answer? I taught this to a young widow I was teaching to coach other widows. She confessed that she actually had problems with deep sadness and depression even before her husband died. Can you image how his death had compounded this for her? After several sessions, I was sincerely praying that something would click for her in understanding that it was her thoughts that were perpetuating these feelings for her. In the fifth week, I taught the class about coaching questions and about asking ourselves a better question. Then I got this note from her:

"Something must have finally clicked after last night's lesson; for the first time EVER in my life, I actually caught myself this morning. While waiting to order a coffee, I became conscious of the question, 'Why am I so unhappy?' playing through my mind. So of course the mind went to work finding answers. But I could change the question and then, therefore, change the focus of the mind! I'm doing cartwheels...."

It is hearing about results like this or seeing the light suddenly come on in the eyes of one of my students that makes coaching so rewarding. Learning to ask a better question was her big breakthrough.

When we are looking to help a client create better results in her life, asking questions that provoke their underlying thoughts is key. I ask questions like:

What are you thinking when you do that?

When that happened, what did you make it mean?

How does it feel when you think that?

What is it you want to be creating in your life?

The answers to these questions are going to be thoughts or feelings. Thoughts are a sentence and a feeling is one word. We are looking to help them create more positive thoughts, and asking the right questions is a powerful way to do that.

A common main question for widows is, "How can I possibly look forward to life without him/her?" The truth, which you want their brain to realize, is, "I can look forward to life again." Change their question to, "How can I begin to enjoy life again?" Suddenly your client will begin to find answers. Whatever the question, decide if it is empowering. If it isn't, help them change it.

Now, there are times when we don't want to feel great, which is also fine. When something tragic happens, like losing a loved one, then you don't want to feel great and that's okay. Let your client know that it is completely okay to choose sadness about her spouse dying. That's not what we're talking about here. We're talking about when she is not feeling great *and* she is not taking responsibility for it. She is blaming it on things outside of herself instead of acknowledging it is her own choice to think the thoughts that make her feel that way.

More ninja coaching questions to ask your client and even ask yourself:

What am I thinking?

Is this thought really true?

Why am I choosing to think this?

Once you've helped your client access their thinking, you can ask them how the thought feels. Help them connect their thoughts to their feelings. Often when we uncover a thought that has been playing in our mind and realize it is not even a little true, we can choose not to think it anymore. It is the awareness of the sentences our brain has been playing that can change us. It is the power of knowing our thoughts are optional and we do not have to believe them any longer. Give this power to your client by helping her see her own thinking and learning how to ask herself a better question!

Chapter 9 – Looking to the Future

Are you stuck in your past? It is a natural thing after losing your spouse to spend a great deal of time looking at the past. As a matter of fact, the mind immediately goes back to that last day to reflect on everything we said, and looks back at the past week and the past month, scanning for anything and everything we may have done wrong. I remember trying to remember all our conversations, thinking, "Did I say I love you? Was I mean to him? Was he mean to me?" This is because in our hearts we want to know we did everything perfectly for them right before they died. It is because we love them so dearly, we cannot bear the thought that we argued or took each other for granted in those final days. Of course, when you allow your brain to scan for all the things you said wrong, it is going to find evidence for you. It is what the brain is programmed to do. Instead, try asking your brain about the loving moments, the moments that felt so secure together that you could take each other's love and commitment to each other for granted. But then, do not allow yourself to stay dreaming in the past.

So many widows who come to me for help are stuck because they keep replaying the past in their mind. There is an old Bill Murray movie called *Groundhog Day*. His character in the film is Phil, a weatherman. He is assigned to do the annual weather news story of the groundhog coming out of his burrow. You know what I'm talking about? All those weird dudes dressed up like pilgrims yanking the poor sleeping groundhog out of his hole to make their proclamation that we are doomed to six more weeks of winter (do they ever give us an early spring?). Anyway, Bill Murray's character gets caught in a blizzard that he should have forecasted. I mean, he is a weatherman after all! As a result, he gets trapped in a time loop, and he is doomed to re-live the same day over and over again until he learns it was not the blizzard that trapped him in reliving the same day, it was how he was reacting to it! This is exactly what happens to us when we keep thinking the same thoughts over and over, day after day.

You see, if our thoughts create our feelings that make us act a certain way and create the results we have in our lives, then if we are thinking the *same thoughts* every day, we are trapped in Groundhog Day. We are living the same day over and over. There comes a time when you need to start thinking new thoughts. There comes a time that you need to begin to look ahead of you to where you are intended to go in your life. You can love your past, treasure the story of your marriage and how that has shaped who you are, and still look forward into the future.

There is nothing in the past that you can actually change. The past cannot reach out to who you are right this second. The only way the past continues to upset you or cause you emotional pain is in the way you are thinking about it. Remember, it is the story you tell yourself that makes the difference. This applies to anything in your past that still causes you emotional trauma. It can only cause you trauma if you choose to think about it in terms of being victimized. We never have to be victims. Our power is in our ability to choose our thoughts.

So when you are working with a widow client, you are going to help her understand this and gently guide her to the understanding that she can and needs to begin considering her new tomorrow. I hear widows all the time say, "But life will never be the same again." Of course, it is not going to be the same. But what they are really trying to say with that statement is, "I will never be as happy, as safe, or as comfortable again." That is a pretty dismal tomorrow to project into the future. This is exactly the Groundhog Day future they've been living and re-living. Instead we want to nudge their focus into what could be different in their tomorrow. What outcomes in their life would they most want to create right now?

Ask your client for her top five outcomes she would love to see in her future. When I ask this in class, I get responses like, "Traveling more, finding a companion just to have dinner or see a movie with, making myself more financially stable, selling our house and moving closer to family, having a career that is more fulfilling so I feel like I'm making a difference in the world." Just beginning to brainstorm on what they would want can begin to make them feel a little excited about the future. It is amazing how few people ever even consider what it is they want! Small wonder people keep plugging away, day after day, in jobs they feel they are going nowhere in, or in relationships that they feel are one-sided. They have never allowed themselves to dream and want something better.

But dreaming is critical for your happiness. Knowing what you want matters, for what you want is the GPS to your destiny. So help your client identify something that she wants that really lights her up when it hits her. As soon as you hear that spark in her voice, you'll know. When she has her list of five things she would want to have in her life, ask her how she spent her days this week. What was her typical day? What did she do yesterday? Here is how most days will look:

I got up and got the kids ready for school.

I dropped the kids off and went to work.

Work was a normal workday, but I was exhausted by the end of it.

I got the kids, got home and helped them get started on homework.

Then I made dinner and after dinner, cleaned up the place.

I got the kids off to bed.

Then I collapsed on the sofa to watch some TV until I went to bed.

Do you see the problem with that day? Not one minute of time was scheduled in to work on a dream for the future. Maybe this client was very lit up by the idea of opening her own healing center or traveling across the US. Yet there was not one step taken toward her future. People are shocked when they acknowledge that they do have a dream, yet do not spend a little time each day working towards that dream! They could be just researching travel routes across the US online after dinner. Maybe check out landmarks they would want to visit along the way. Begin mapping hotels. No matter they do not have the funds for it or the time off for it. If they never take any steps, it will never happen.

Helping your client know what she wants for herself (not for her kids or for her other family members – for *her*) is important for her ability to recover from the deep sadness of loss. It can be just one small dream. In one of my classes, a widow who wanted to get out more began visiting all the beautiful libraries in her area that she could drive to on a day trip. She loved libraries and her area in California had some amazing libraries. It was not traveling to Europe, as she first described, that changed her life and her outlook, but rather taking a weekly day trip to another new library. It was starting small on that dream of travel, and it was breaking her away from Groundhog Day!

Chapter 10 – How to Get Things Done

Widows often feel that they will never have dreams of the future again. Your client may feel deep guilt when she turns her thoughts to her dreams because she has believed that being widowed means you have to stay in sadness forever. Our culture portrays "good widows" only in a state of mourning. It may feel to your client like she is not honoring her husband's death if she feels happy and excited about the future. It is the rare widow who sees the opposite to be true. Once widows realize that not only can they dream again and plan for the future, it is admirable to step back into life and celebrate the memory of their husband, they are ready to let go of depression and look ahead. Then you can begin to help her lay out a plan to work toward a dream or even just be able to complete a project.

With the foggy brain we all experience through the first year of widowhood, it is very difficult to remain focused on any task. You can coach your client around her thoughts that she cannot possibly get anything done. Helping your client understand the thinking that has held her back from the results she wants in her life is your number one job as a coach. The cause is always in our thinking. But there are also great techniques to learn and share, once her thoughts around accomplishing something are cleaned up.

Start with a brainstorming session. Ask your client to list 25 things she wants. These can be objects. They can be how she wants to feel. If she is having trouble with this task and feels resistance to it, it is a perfect opportunity to start asking her why and get down to the thoughts she is having about wanting things. It is important to want things in our life. We need to have wants for personal growth, tangible items, and even spiritual connection. She can list anything she wants. When you help her understand her limiting thoughts and feelings about the exercise, she will find it fun once she gets started writing her list.

After her list is written, it is interesting to discuss and ask her if she included anything on her list that she already has. This is powerful. Help her acknowledge the things she has in her life right now that she wants. Her home? Her job? Her beautiful kids? It is important that we want the things we already have and love having. So if you love the car you have, then you continue to want it. It is powerful energy when you can come from a feeling of abundance and gratitude for things you already have when you are thinking about things you would like to have. I know it sounds a little "out there," but truly you want to be creating a feeling of abundance and having when you dream of what you want. When you want something from a space of "it would be nice, but …" or, "I couldn't really afford this …" it holds you back from being able to create that very thing in your life. All you are putting out in your mind is a sense of lacking that thing instead of actually being able to have the thing. If you are dreaming of something you think you can never have, it actually causes emotional pain. We are dreaming of it because we don't have it and the dreaming is reminding us that we don't have it. Widows and widowers stop dreaming because they don't want that contrast; they don't want to think about what they want versus the loss they have suffered.

So now, help your client rewrite her list to include some things she already has that she does want. Her list might include her house because she loves it and feels gratitude that she has that house. Intermingle those things she already has as wants with the wants that are not in her life yet. Help her feel that the things she wants are reachable. She is now wanting from a place of *having*. That changes the mood and energy. It is not underscoring what she does not have. It tricks the mind and thus shifts the emotional energy of it.

It can be helpful at this point to have your client write out a dream to-do list. This is a thought download of big dreams, little tasks that she is wanting to tackle, crazy ideas – even hidden desires. She needs to just start writing as quickly as she can every item that pops into her head. Set a timer for no more than two minutes for her to write as quickly as she can. She can compare her to-do list with the wants she wrote out in the first exercise. Have her narrow down her lists to the five things she feels are the most important. These are her top five priorities of what she wants. Now they can begin to feel more concrete. She can write them in a current, positive fashion. Instead of "I want to go visit France," she needs to write, "I am going to visit France." Make it real. Make it as if it is inevitable, because then it becomes inevitable. Ask her to reflect on what she did in her life yesterday and the day before that. Were her actions in line with the priorities on her list? What can she change in her daily life to better align with the things she wants? It is amazing how we can wish for something, but never take even 15 minutes out of our daily life to put toward researching and creating that thing! It just never even enters our consciousness that we could be working toward something that felt "unreachable" to us.

Your client can take any one of her goals and list all the things she would need to do in order to achieve it. Have her go into great detail and list every possible step. Then you can have her figure out how much time each step would take, and then even schedule the steps in her calendar. If she commits to doing each step on the day it is listed on her calendar with no exceptions, then it is going to be inevitable that she will accomplish what she felt was impossible. All those small tasks that she came to you saying she could not possibly focus on and complete since becoming widowed suddenly are completely doable and on her calendar. If she schedules out steps to finish something in four weeks, those four weeks will go by with all the little steps being done – and suddenly, her task is accomplished like magic. She only needs to dedicate a bit of her time each day to working on the one piece of the puzzle. It is no longer something overwhelming because she is looking at the end game of what she needs to do. Learning how to do this will change her life. Teaching yourself how to do this will change your life!

Chapter 11 – When That Inner Child Shows Up

Children do not have a fully developed prefrontal cortex in their brains. That actually takes a number of years to grow and develop in human beings! But there is a good reason for this. As children, our brains need to be open to everything around us and readily absorb it all. It is why we begin to struggle to stand up and walk around the age of one. We've been seeing this demonstrated by the grownups around us and with our child mind, we never question that this is supposed to be us, too. Children learn at an accelerated rate because of this completely open brain. With this open brain, children will assume that everything that they feel and experience is coming from outside of them. It is the mechanism of that rapid learning and growth. Ever watch a child struggle to put on their own shoe, only to throw the shoe down in frustration and say, "dumb shoe"? To them, it is not their own limitations preventing them from putting on the shoe. It is the shoe's fault. Everything that happens to the child is coming from outside them. It is all happening *to them.*

Eventually around the age of 23 years old, the prefrontal cortex is completed. When I first learned that the prefrontal cortex of the brain was not fully formed until then, I thought, "Well, that explains a lot about my early twenties." It is the very rational area of our brain where we can make good decisions for ourselves by being able to compare one thing to another. We can think about our own thoughts in the prefrontal cortex. We are the only animal (as far as I know) who can think about their own thoughts. It makes us human. Yes, we do begin to compare one thing to another before the age of 23 (at least I seem to remember making some choices, though they were not all good ones), but the ability is not completed.

Here's the kicker; most adults are still functioning like they did as little kids. I'm not saying they are immature in all ways. I'm saying that they still think that everything they feel is happening *to them*, not by them. They think everything is coming from outside of them! You'll hear this when they are blaming their boss for everything, blaming their job for their stress, blaming their friend, blaming the government, blaming the economy, on and on. They not only blame outside factors for how they feel, they even blame things outside of them for how they act and the results this creates in their lives!

It is not their fault. There was no course in high school to teach us about our thoughts and feelings. There is no course required for graduation that covers emotional adulthood. This is a terrible way to live your life because you think everything you feel and everything that happens to you is beyond your control. It is not. It is all completely within your control. You have a prefrontal cortex that can look at your own thoughts, how those thoughts are making you feel and act. You can choose to think differently. Instead of pointing a finger outside of you, you can instead take responsibility and choose how you want to think and feel. Only you can correct course because you surely cannot control the people and things around you.

So what does it mean to be an emotional adult? It means that you take responsibility both for your pain and for your joy. You know that it is the thought you choose to focus on that creates those emotions. You don't expect other people to *make* you happy. That could be a long wait, my friend. Instead you take responsibility for your own happiness by learning how to create that emotion for yourself. You can understand and appreciate that you are the only one who can hurt your feelings – you do this with the thoughts you are thinking.

Now as you begin to help your widow clients understand this, it is not going to be immediate or easy for them to change. It is a big undertaking to strive for emotional adulthood, but it is going to be the single most rewarding task of their life. You will be teaching your client that she is not at the mercy of other people or at the mercy of circumstances. If she blames her mother-in-law for hurting her, she is giving her mother-in-law that power. Help her see that she is handing over responsibility for her feelings to her mother-in-law (or friend, or boss, or whoever she is blaming how she feels on). Would she really want them in charge of her emotions? No, of course not!

Once you teach this to your client and she begins working on emotional adulthood, do not let her think that she is going to react in that adult mode always and never falter. We all revert back into emotional childhood on occasion. We want to throw our shoes and yell and toss ourselves down onto the ground. But when you can recognize it in yourself, you have the opportunity to redirect your thoughts.

When do I experience emotional childhood? Oh, dear – in the car, driving, especially in traffic. I find myself saying "Come on, *come on!*" It never fails to make me laugh when I hear myself do that. I recognize that little girl still living inside of me immediately. She's the one who threw her crayons across our family room because they would not stay neatly inside the lines while I colored. But the bonus is that I can spot her right away, laugh at myself, and course correct. I know full well that I am at no time a victim. Help your client understand this, too. She is not a victim of her circumstances. She can completely take hold of those feelings and choose to feel and act differently. When we can do this, it feels so much better and creates much better outcomes in our lives.

Chapter 12 – Others Don't Live Up to Our Expectations

If you are a widow coach, expect to hear a lot about how others are behaving or not behaving. There is always the complaint about friends who disappear after we become widowed. This is unfortunately true. Friends will say, "I'm so sorry for your loss. Let me know if there's anything you need." Then they promptly disappear, permanently. But even more distressing to your clients will be family members who do not act as expected. You'll hear about employers who do not act as expected. The widow is very hurt by the way others are acting in her life. But here's the thing; people will always be just who they are. They get to do that. You get to be just who you are too. You get to act exactly as you choose to. No one else can "make" you be something different. You cannot make them be different, either, and it is only going to frustrate you to no end when you try.

All this difficulty comes from the manuals we carry around with us in our heads. It is an instruction guide we have for someone in our life about how we would like them to act so we can feel good and be happy. No one else even knows we have a manual for them, but we do, and we know every single page by heart. Perhaps you have a page in your friend manual that says a friend should always return your phone calls promptly. Or a page that says when you become widowed, your friend should respond to your needs immediately. You have a sister manual that says your sister should invite you to every party she ever throws. How dare she have a dinner for friends and not let you know? You have this written right on page three of the sister manual in your head! We begin to believe that we could be so much happier if our friend, sister, coworkers would all just behave as we expect them to. We are pinning our happiness on others instead of taking responsibility for making ourselves happy. We are giving all our power away to others by writing those instructions in our mental manuals.

The manual is a concept that first shocks my widow clients because they can immediately recognize all the expectations they have for others. They are going to want to defend their expectations! They are going to tell you why all their manual instructions are completely reasonable. But what you are going to teach them is how those manuals only serve to make them unhappy because you cannot manipulate others into doing and acting exactly as we wish. Nor would your widow client want those other people trying to manipulate her!

The best manual example is going to be the manual she had for her spouse. I can remember that my manual said that Jim should automatically take out the garbage after dinner without bitching about it. Period. It was *his job*. Right? I always did all the cleaning and organizing in the household. He could at least just do the garbage every evening and not stomp around and ask, "Why do I always have to take out the garbage? How do you make so much garbage?" This was a daily irritation for years, for both of us. Finally, after more than a decade of this, I realized it would be so much easier if I just grabbed the stupid garbage bag toward the end of cooking dinner and walked it the five steps across the porch to the garbage can. Then I didn't have to hear the whining.

Okay, I know – it all sounds less than gracious. You see, at that time, I had not fully understood that we all carry around a husband manual. But it did start to sink into my brain that I was trying to force him to do something he didn't want to and that was not fun for either of us. It was amazing. Suddenly all the friction over the garbage stopped. Some evenings he would even just come by and grab the garbage without saying a word. Some evenings I would get it. It was no longer a big deal. We no longer groused at each other about it. What a stupid rule in my husband manual that had us at odds right at dinner time! Now dinner was more enjoyable together. I let go of one little expectation and it changed our evenings together.

So ask your client what was in her husband manual. Can she see this in hindsight? With that knowledge, what is in her sister/friend/mother manual right now that is making her so unhappy? Can she acknowledge it is her manual? She is trying to force someone to behave in a way that serves her instead of them. Help her understand that if she can just rip that page out of her manual, she is going to be so much happier. Better yet, burn that entire manual. Trying to manipulate others never works and only serves to create friction. There is nothing you ever have to do in your life, and there is nothing anyone else has to do for you. Ask her how she feels if she is in a relationship where she is expected to be a certain way that goes against who she is? Would she want to be responsible for someone else feeling happy 100% of the time? If she expects others to make her happy, she is going to be constantly disappointed. Most other people in her life are having enough trouble making their selves happy. If she has a friend who is constantly needy, she will agree that it is not much fun to be around that person. When two people are both taking responsibility for their own happiness, they can get together and have fun. This is what builds amazing relationships.

Helping your client see the manual she has for someone who she says has been upsetting her is the first step in her being able to let go of that manual. Begin to explore with your client what it is she wants other people to do differently and why. The answer is always going to be if the other person changed, then your client could feel better. But remember, her feelings do not come from outside of her. It is her thoughts that create her feelings, not the other person. So the truth that you are teaching is that her feelings do not depend on what the other person is doing. The other person doing something that follows her manual does not mean that they love and care for her. Not following her manual does not mean that they don't love or care for her! Feeling loved and cared for comes from our thoughts about the other person, not from our expectations of them. When she can stop trying to control the other person (or people) in her life, it will be a huge relief. Just like grabbing that kitchen garbage yourself and walking it across the porch. When you can help your client embrace this, it sets them up for happy, long-lasting, and conflict-free relationships.

Chapter 13 – Loving "Just Because"

As widows, we feel a lot of loneliness and deep sadness. We are missing out on a lot of love. But that love was not coming from outside of us, so it cannot truly be taken away from us. Remember, how you feel comes from the sentences your mind plays for you. It was all the thoughts that you had about your spouse that made you feel loved. It was not the things he said, but what you thought about the things he said. It was not the things he did, but what you thought about the things he did.

A widowed client Pat told me about how her husband's ex-wife showed up at the funeral. They had been divorced for decades, yet here she was all dressed in black. It was not just that she showed up that had Pat fit to be tied. It was the fact that she showed up in full grief and drama making a large show of this. Now, I'm sure you remember how you felt immediately after the death of your spouse. There was such shock you could not even cry and grieve initially. I know it was a couple of days before I cried because I was like a walking zombie. At the funeral, you most likely tried to buck up and just get through it. But now here came Pat's husband's former spouse, as Pat described it, "in full Hollywood display of grieving widow." To make Pat feel even angrier, mutual friends all rushed to the ex's side to console her, leaving Pat standing in a "receiving line." All this had actually happened almost a year prior to when I was coaching Pat, yet Pat still burned and seethed over this. It caused her a lot of distress just relaying the story to me. She had not relayed the story to many others because she didn't want to sound petty and it frankly felt humiliating to her. So you can imagine Pat's face when I suggested she could feel love for the ex-wife instead. She was immediately saying, "Are you kidding? Why would I ever feel love for her?" I asked, "Why don't you want to feel love when you think of her? Why don't you want to feel that emotion?" It was obvious it hadn't even occurred to her that it was even an option to feel love toward her husband's ex. She had lots of reasons why she "shouldn't feel love." She was feeling terrible every time she had to be around her and using the ex-wife's actions at the funeral as a reason for her to feel terrible. But what she was really doing was giving all of her emotional power away to the ex-wife and experiencing negative emotion. Instead of taking responsibility for her feelings, she was blaming her feelings on the ex-wife. I explained to her that she can feel however she wants toward her.

When you explain to someone that love is an option, and you're talking about someone they don't even like, they tend to think, "What are you talking about? I don't want to love someone I don't like. I don't even like them. Why would I want to love them?" But the reason is because you get to feel that emotion. You get to feel love when you love someone. The really good news is the other person doesn't get it, right? Just because you love her doesn't mean it jumps into her body, and she gets to experience it. You are the only one feeling it, just like you're the only one feeling the hate. She doesn't feel your hate. She feels her own emotion, and you get to feel yours.

My client Pat initially said she could just feel neutral toward the ex-wife. That is what she felt she could "compromise" with. But my answer was, "Why would you choose 'neutral' when feeling love feels so much better inside?" Thoughts always vibrate from your mind into your body as feelings. There is scientific evidence of this. The brain releases the chemicals and hormones that create emotions. For example, the brain chemicals of dopamine, oxytocin, serotonin, and endorphins all activate feelings of happiness. Brain scans of young lovers show that dopamine and norepinephrine production light up. Dr. Helen Fisher found that the caudate nucleus (a part of the lower brain) is highly activated. The mere presence of another individual cannot cause such changes in your body, but what you are thinking about them does.

For sure, by now, you know where I'm going with this. If it is our thoughts that trigger feelings of love and being loved, then we can choose to feel this any time we want. Isn't that amazing? Think about how wonderful it feels to love someone. Remember what it felt like when you first fell in love. Can you conjure up that wonderful, butterflies, walking- on-air, feeling? I bet you can. Feeling love, just like any other emotion we experience, is a matter of choice. If we could choose to feel love, why wouldn't we?

Conversely, feeling hate or any variation of hate is also based on your thoughts and the neuroscience cascade those thoughts set in motion. Feeling hate does *absolutely nothing* to the person you are feeling this emotion toward. It does not jump from your body into theirs to punish them. The only thing hate does is make you feel terrible. So what if... what if you could choose to turn hate around into love – every time? Sound challenging? Oh, yes, it is – until you begin to build evidence in your life of this working out for you. Will the other person suddenly be rewarded with your love? Nope. Just like hating them does not actually punish them, loving them for who they are does not jump out of your body to reward them. It rewards you.

This is unconditional love. You can choose this every day of your life. It may not be as easy as it was to feel love when your spouse was around, but you still get to have it. Loving unconditionally does not mean that you have to condone terrible behavior on the part of another person. Pat did not need to approve of the ex-wife's behavior at the funeral. But after coaching and pondering what the ex could have been thinking, Pat began to come around to realizing how much the ex-wife must have been hurting all those decades, and how awful her husband's ex was choosing to make herself feel that day with the thoughts she was not only thinking, but also expressing. Pat could even begin to feel a little compassion for what the ex was creating in her own life.

You can fall in love with every person you meet. Seriously! I was in line at the grocery store one afternoon and the person in front of me was taking way too long for their transactions to be completed. I found myself starting to feel impatient and even seethe a bit. As soon as I caught myself feeling that way, I realized I could instead feel some compassion and even start to fall in love with the checker. He was a very young man, clearly new on the job. So as I stepped over after he finished with a particular difficult transaction, I gave him a warm smile. We joked back and forth a bit as he rang up my purchases, and by the time my bags were in my cart, I was totally in love with this kid. I wanted to adopt him. Of course, I could not exactly lean across the counter and say, "I just love you." How creepy would that have been? But I smiled all the way to my car, realizing I had turned my impatience right around to a wonderful feeling of loving on someone else. That lightness in my heart and in my step lasted the entire afternoon! Every person I encountered on the rest of my errands benefited from the warm smile I was carrying with me. Nothing could drag me back down!

The client who came to me for weight loss and also suspected her husband was cheating on her did not realize that continuing to love him anyway was option. She automatically assumed if he were cheating she would have to leave her home and give up on him. Even worse, what she made it all mean was that he should not bother loving her because she was overweight. She felt she was not at all lovable or worth being loved. Being loveable is something that comes from inside of us. It is not what someone else sees in us. Loveable is love-ABLE. It is our ability to *be loved*. When you can reach the place where you are able to love no matter what, you are building on your ability to be loved. This client was making herself miserable with all her thoughts and stories about her husband. The point was not even whether he was really having an affair or not. I was not there to coach her husband. Manipulating your husband's behavior is not possible (and oh yeah, husbands just love it when someone is trying to manipulate them). The place where change could begin was in my client's thoughts of unworthiness. Her story about what was going on with her husband could be rewritten by her. When she began looking at all her thoughts around her story of what was happening with her husband, she started to see how much of what she had been thinking was not absolutely true. It was thoughts she was choosing to think and painful assumptions she was making. She indeed felt love for her husband, but the unconditional love she needed to learn and feel was for *herself.*

If you do not feel love, this is not a reason to beat yourself up and make yourself now feel guilty on top of not feeling love! Just ask yourself why you are choosing to not feel love in that moment. If you are making it be all about the person and not wanting them to be rewarded for abominable behavior, remember that it is an emotion that you get to feel privately. It makes you feel good. By no means do you need to call your husband's ex to tell her you love her (although that would be pretty awesome if you think about it!). Unconditional love is the ultimate gift you can give yourself. You will treat yourself better when you are feeling love!

As a widow who missed feeling loved acutely after my husband died, I have learned the luxury of allowing myself to feel love at every given opportunity. I fall in love over and over. My favorite way to wrap up my class on unconditional love for my certified widow coaches is to tell them all, "I love all of you and there is nothing you can do about it!"

Chapter 14 – Why We All Need an Outside Perspective

Now that you've gotten this far through the book and have been introduced to many of the concepts I teach as a coach, your mind might be reeling a bit with the amount of information and insight. It takes a lot of hands-on practice and guidance to really integrate these tools into your life and apply them to helping others. Your best practice is going to be coaching yourself. I had been told once that therapists are required to undergo psychotherapy as part of their training. Sadly, I later discovered this is not true in the United States. It surely should be required. You cannot understand the impact of coaching until you have been coached. You cannot come to a session with a client without having coached your own mind to clear any pre-judgement or expectations of working with that client.

An intensive part of my training as a certified life coach was being coached by other coaches and learning to coach myself, all in addition to learning how to coach others. Over the years since that time, I have self-coached on a daily basis. Managing your mind is a little like cleaning house. You can do a really good, deep cleaning, but that does not mean you will never have to clean again. I have also hired and worked with other coaches, especially when I needed an outside perspective on an issue that I could not get my arms around. Over and over I hear coaches saying, "Even life coaches need coaches." This is the truth. Most daily issues and emotions I can self-coach around. But occasionally I hit a rock in the road that I circle and circle without being able to figure out why it is driving me into emotional spin. That is when I reach out to my coach. When you are inside the bottle, you cannot possibly read the label on the front of the bottle yourself.

It is one thing to read about these tools and concepts of coaching, but it is an entirely different experience to work in a class and begin to implement them in your life. Watching another coach in action and how these concepts and tools are applied when working with an actual widow client takes it to another level. Is it worth taking the time to apply all this to your own life? It most definitely is worth the time and the work. Understanding your own innermost workings and thoughts is the work of our lives. I believe it is why we are here.

But trying to go it alone is not going to work. You need to surround yourself with other widow coaches, a group of peers, to continue to inspire you and challenge you. I love keeping my classes small so the students in my class can connect. They become very close and open with each other. They bond over the weeks of learning and graduate with their own "posse" of widow coaches to stay in close contact with and continue advanced learning together. It's like knives against steel – the associations continually sharpen each other. Without my own coaches that I have learned alongside over the years, it would be a lonely profession indeed! We constantly challenge each other to stretch our skills and reach even higher potential as coaches.

Learning to create my own business after a life of working for others has been quite challenging, but also the most amazing adventure of my life. The coaches I've hired to help with my business as a life coach have made a huge impact on both my life and business. It has been pure pleasure to work with every one of them. My life over the last three years has now entirely changed. I continue to hold very dear the 21 years I was blessed to have with Jim and all that I learned with him. Now I celebrate where I've taken all that and who I've become, and I'm hoping he is where he can peek in on my life and cheer me on. I know how excited he must be if he is.

I could not do it alone, even though I work as a lone entrepreneur and am alone most of the time in my work. It is the associates I have through my business, my fellow coaches that I continue to journey forward alongside, the coaches I've hired, and most especially widows I'm honored to teach and work with that have filled my life with excitement and immense joy. It all started with taking the huge, terrifying step of deciding this is what I wanted to do with the rest of my life, paying for training at a time I was worried about even buying a new lipstick, and then standing up tall and going *all in*. "All in" meant that I was committed to becoming the best life coach I could be. I would not have succeeded without the learning and the connections I made along the way while becoming certified as a coach. Certification makes a tremendous difference, not only in your credibility as a widow coach, but in the process and the impact that path will have on your life. Even if you think, like so many of my students do, you will never really do anything with your widow coach certification, I encourage you to take the leap and go get certified as a coach. You just may surprise yourself!

Chapter 15 – In Conclusion

So even as you begin to practice and learn what is in this book about coaching, find some connection and support outside of your own desk and chair. Continue to stretch and learn coaching concepts. There are widows out there trying to find someone to connect with who can understand them. Only a widow can truly understand and coach another widow. I say this over and over again because it is truth. This is an experience unlike any other loss or grief you will experience in your life.

According to the U.S. Bureau of the Census in 1999, "Nearly 700,000 women lose their husbands each year and will be widows for an average of 14 years." The census of 1999 is the most recent statistic for the number of widows in the United States. It showed 13.6 million widows at that time. I can only imagine how that number has grown since then. The majority of these 13.6 million women are feeling like no one understands, not their family, not their friends, not the counselor they saw, not even the therapist they hired. They are waiting for a widow coach. I realized I could never reach over 13 million widows, until it dawned on me what is needed in the world is widow coaches in every community. This is why I set out to begin instructing and certifying widow coaches. Much to my surprise, I saw that the class created more, far more, than I ever expected. The transformations I was seeing in my clients taking the class were amazing and the direction their lives would go surprised us all.

So just like it was entirely up to us to pick up the shattered pieces around us when our life partners died, it is up to us to now reach out a hand to those who are still lost among the shards. You can learn and practice a new way of understanding how to process your emotions and manage your thoughts to create the results you want in your life. On your path as a widow coach, you will be able to help others to discover the truth of their own thoughts and help them ease the emotional pain that has plagued them. You will change the life of every widow you coach. Are you ready? Are you all in? Step forward, widow coach.

Further Reading

Widowed, by Joann Filomena

The Power of Intention: Learning to Co-create Your World Your Way, by Dr. Wayne W. Dyer

The Top Ten Things Dead People Want to Tell You, by Mike Dooley

Illusions: The Adventures of a Reluctant Messiah, by Richard Bach

Oprah's Saving Gracie, by Oprah Winfrey, *O Magazine* August 2007 Issue

What Doesn't Kill Us: The New Psychology of Posttraumatic Growth, by Stephen Joseph

Awaken the Giant Within, Tony Robbins

Acknowledgments

It has been my honor to teach widows the tools I've used in the way I've developed them to help widows live an extraordinary life. They freely opened their hearts to me and in the process of becoming certified widow coaches, found their own future again. Without them, this book could not have been written. So thank you to each and every widow that has come through my class.

Of course, none of this would have happened without some amazing mentors who have become a part of my life along the way. Special thanks to Brooke Castillo, CEO of The Life Coach School, for giving so freely of herself to her coaches and to the world. Brooke continues to serve as an amazing example of what is possible in my work and in my life. It was the tools of life coaching that helped me move forward in my new life.

Thanks to Angela Lauria, Publisher at Difference Press, for always being at my back, inspiring new goals and new confidence in what I can create in the world. When I toyed with the idea of a second book for widows who want to learn coaching, Angela was right there to say, "I'd endorse that book right this second. Write it." Thank you, Angela, for your unwavering belief in my inner author.

Lastly, and as always, I want to thank my greatest mentor and teacher for over 20 years who gave me the gift of who I am today: Jim Filomena. Though Jim passed from this reality almost three years ago now, there remains so much of him and his influences in my life. Together we explored how our thoughts created our reality, and now, today, I teach this very premise. Joann The Life Coach would have never existed if it were not for all those years of shared books, tapes, discussions, adventures, and mad, crazy love.

Love, Joann

About the Author

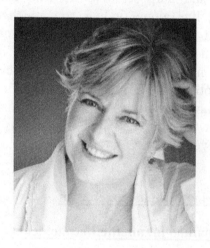

Professional Certified Life Coach Joann Filomena teaches widows how to coach widows, so they both gain meaning in their lives again. Joann resides in the heart of the beautiful Hudson Valley; she is the producer and host of "Widow Cast," "Weight Coach," and "*This is Us* Podcast," with listeners spanning the globe. Joann uses her life experience and coaching skills to help numerous clients through widowhood, weight loss, and many other life issues that arise in those sessions with incredible authenticity and compassion.

As a life coach, she has seen profound,

extraordinary transformations in the lives of her clients and students. The new widow who felt all her life plans pulled out from under her on the death of her husband, now moving ahead in her life with direction and purpose. Widows who feared they could not live alone finding how much they can savor and thrive in their very own space. The widow who could not even get out of bed most mornings now looks forward to each new day of reaching others in her practice as a certified widow coach. Joann constantly reminds us all that we can move forward after loss into tremendous personal growth, even as we carry those we've lost in our hearts.

Website: <u>joannthelifecoach.com</u>

Email: <u>Joann@joannethelifecoach.com</u>

Facebook:
<u>www.facebook.com/joannthelifecoach/</u>

Widow Coaches Class: <u>widowcoaches.com</u>

Thank You

Thank you for reading *The Widow Coach*.

As a special thank you, I invite you to the replay of my online workshop I created to share the first lesson I teach in Widow Coaches Class. Just go to this link and enter your email address so I can get it to you: **Joannbooks.com**

I'd love to hear about your journey through widowhood. Please email me or comment on Facebook on the page for the *Widow Cast* podcast: **www.facebook.com/widowcast/**

My email is Joann@JoannTheLifeCoach.com
Visit my website at JoannTheLifeCoach.com

Last but certainly not least, I invite you to download and listen to my podcast for widows. I had always loved listening to podcasts, so it was no surprise that after my spouse passed, I went searching in iTunes to hear something, anything from another widow. At that time, there was not one podcast for widows. It was in my heart to do this podcast and a year later, I made it a reality. It is free to download, listen, subscribe! **joannthelifecoach.com/widowcast**

Made in the USA
Coppell, TX
22 July 2020

31350985R00059